Gluten Free Club: Gluten-Free Made Simple Curb Fatigue, Reduce Inflammation, Lose Weight

By Shari Darling
www.understandpublishing.com

Special Thanks to my Editor,

Deanna Shanti, Shanti Publishing

About the Author

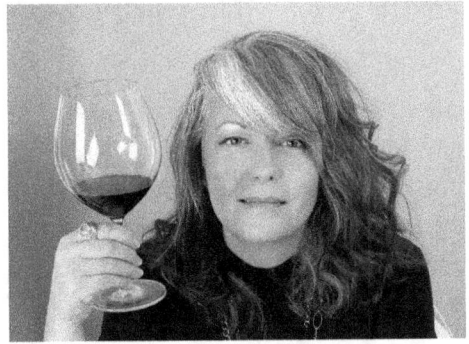

Hi, my name is Shari Darling.

I am a food and wine cookbook author, newspaper columnist, wine judge, restaurant reviewer and educator of wine and food. My website is **http://sharidarling.com**

Quite by accident I discovered a few years ago that I am gluten-sensitive. At first I thought this discovery would hamper my work in wine and food. This is not the case at all.

I call this guidebook "Gluten-Free Diet – Made Simple" because going Gluten-Free does not require you to cut portions or count calories. It is not about starving your body of fats or carbohydrates. It is also not about weighing your food or removing bananas. It's mostly about eating a generally healthy diet of whole foods and finding substitutions to enjoy the foods you've always loved. Eat bread, just choose a Gluten-Free version and eat in moderation. Enjoy pasta? Then eat pasta, but find a decent Gluten-Free version and eat in moderation. The only strict rule is to avoid boxed and pre-prepared Gluten-Free foods.

I am not advocating that everyone must be on a Gluten-Free diet. I don't think wheat is bad. However, having read a plethora of books on the subject of wheat and Gluten-Free and having experienced the benefits of Gluten-Free first hand, I can honestly say it's the best choice for me and for anyone else who is experiencing side effects from gluten. I can tell you that a Gluten-Free diet has greatly contributed to both my husband and I shedding unwanted pounds. It's not the only contributor.

We eat a healthy diet, watch food portions, drink alcohol moderately and exercise regularly as well. But going Gluten-Free really is super simple.

I discovered my gluten sensitivity after an evening of entertaining Gluten-Free friends. When entertaining I like to cater to my friends' specific culinary diets and requirements. I enjoy the challenge of meeting their dietary needs and surprising them with specialized, multi course meals paired with complementary wines.

About 4 years ago I decided to have a girlfriend and her husband over for a multi-course meal. My girlfriend is gluten- intolerant. So for the main entree I made homemade Gluten-Free lasagna accompanied by Gluten-Free garlic bread.

I had prepared enough lasagna for 12 people, hoping to wrap up the leftovers to give to my girlfriend to take home with her. We all enjoyed the lasagna so much we emptied the over-sized baking dish. When over-indulging on pasta and bread, I expect to wake up the next morning feeling hung-over, face and stomach bloated. I normally arise at 6 a.m. But after an evening of pasta I expect to wake up much later, closer to 8 am. It has always been this way. I have tolerated the effects of pasta and bread on my digestive system, believing the side effects came from the fact that pasta and bread are carbohydrates that makes everyone groggy.

The morning after this particular lasagna indulgence I woke up at 6:30 am and felt surprisingly alert. My stomach felt and looked flat and empty and was at peace. No grumbling. My face was normal, not bloated. This was the beginning of my awakening to the fact that I may have been gluten-sensitive.

I started eating Gluten-Free foods sporadically, not wanting to give up my love of pasta made with semolina flour and my addiction to all kinds of bread. But over time and with supermarkets implementing a whole section of Gluten-Free products, I started to eat Gluten-Free more often. For some time now I have been completely Gluten-Free. I have dropped those extra pounds and feel great.

My brother Jay has finally identified the link between his legs swelling after drinking wheat beer. Two other members of our immediate family suffer from chronic and debilitating irritable bowel syndrome, arthritis and migraines.

In a family of six members, 4 of us suffer from symptoms related to gluten-intolerance. Celiac disease is a genetically predisposed, hereditary condition. Gluten-sensitivity (non celiac) is in an estimated 30% of the population. New research indicates that gluten-sensitivity or intolerance is gene-related to some degree.

I personally believe our family issues have less to do with genetics and more to do with our overconsumption of wheat, barley and rye in its many forms. I go into more detail regarding wheat further on.

My husband suffers from dementia and arthritis. He recently embraced a Gluten-Free diet, has lost weight and is suffering less joint pain. Through research to slow the progression of this deadly disease of dementia I discovered a book called Grain Brain – The Surprising Truth about Wheat, Carbs, and Sugar – Your Brain's Silent Killers. A renowned neurologist Dr. David Perlmutter wrote Grain Brain.

In his book, Dr. Perlmutter explains what happens when the brain encounters common ingredients in our daily bread and fruit bowls and why the brain actually requires more fat and cholesterol, which can spur the growth of new brain cells at any age. With a revolutionary 4-week plan, GRAIN BRAIN teaches us how we can reprogram our genetic destiny for the better.

Given this diagnosis, I converted Jack to a Gluten-Free diet as well. Now we both enjoy interesting and delicious Gluten-Free meals that are healthy. He used to visit Tim Horton's every morning for an Everything Bagel with Herbed Cream Cheese. Now he toasts a Gluten-Free bagel at home and smothers it in homemade cream cheese. You can easily make homemade fresh cheeses (like cream cheese, ricotta, mozzarella, mascarpone) to enjoy that are lower in fat and calories. The Internet is filled with recipes. And once you taste fresh cream cheese or fresh ricotta or mozzarella, chances are, like me, you'll never go back to store bought versions.

In moving to Gluten-Free foods, Jack has lost weight and is suffering less joint pain. He did not care, nor did he notice at first. But it was others who took notice and said, "Jack you've lost weight. You look amazing." These comments inspired Jack to remain on his Gluten-Free diet. Now he has pulled in his belt buckle by more than 2 inches! And he understands why remaining on a Gluten-Free diet is beneficial for his brain.

I share my discoveries in the Gluten-Free Club on Facebook:

http://theglutenfreeclub.net/facebook

I advocate that a Gluten-Free diet can benefit everyone who is interested in healing the body and brain.

A Gluten-Free diet can be a beneficial choice to help anyone lose weight, providing it is embraced in a healthy way. It's not just about eliminating gluten from your diet. It means cooking at home more often and avoiding boxed and refined processed foods – even if they are Gluten-Free. Processed Gluten-Free foods often lack important minerals, vitamins and fiber and are made with substitute starches such as rice and tapioca flour that really have no nutritional value at all. And worse, these products have high glycemic indexes, and sometimes higher fat and sugar. Gluten-Free is not healthier if you consume processed foods.

Avoiding bread and pasta is also not enough and it's really not necessary. Gluten-Free bread and pasta consumed in moderation will help you sustain this lifestyle. There's no need to sacrifice.

Be a conscious shopper. Read labels. Gluten is used in countless products. It is used in soups, gravies, vinaigrettes, sauces, cereals, teas, coffee, spices and so on. It is important to read labels; gluten content can be difficult to spot. Labels might feature ingredients that you may not recognize -- ingredients with gluten-related scientific names. Or an item might contain an ingredient that possesses gluten, of which you are unaware, such as bulgur, couscous, farina, and malt.

A Gluten-Free diet requires an emphasis on consuming fresh produce and avoiding foods containing wheat, barley and rye. Getting sound nutrition is key, along with 8 hours of quality sleep, consuming lots of distilled water (water in its purest form), undertaking regular exercise and surrounding oneself with caring family and friends. Surround yourself with people who inspire you to be your best.

I've developed this guide to give you access to the possibility of healing your body, mind and spirit and the possibility of shedding those unwanted pounds.

I am not a doctor. I am a Gluten-Free consumer. This e-book simply provides some simple and best practices, advice, tips and food suggestions I've obtained through my own gluten-sensitivity journey. Take what ideas work for you and be sure to consult your doctor.

To support you in your journey and to check out our other books in this genre and others go to Understand Publishing and click the icon called "Our Books".

Table of Contents

CHAPTER ONE: Introduction: What is Gluten-Free?

I want to thank you and congratulate you for purchasing the book, "Gluten-Free Made Simple: Curb Fatigue, Reduce Inflammation, Lose Weight."

This book contains information, tips, steps and strategies on how to successfully live a Gluten-Free lifestyle, potentially heal your body from ailments and provide you with the inspiration and possibility of losing weight.

In choosing to open this book, you've taken the first step to creating a healthier and possibly slimmer you! Remember, it's not the information in this guide that will have you lose weight. It is what you utilize from this guide that will make the difference.

The Gluten-Free diet is not about deprivation. You'll lose weight on a Gluten-Free diet IF you do it the right way. If you do it the wrong way, those extra pounds will cling to your hips, stomach and thighs. And in fact, you can gain weight if you get lazy in your food choices.

And remember, even at your current weight, there is nothing wrong with you. You are perfect just the way you are.

Losing weight is about embracing the concepts of patience and discipline. In my teens, 20's and 30's I worked out excessively. I cared only about how I looked, not about how healthy I was. By my 40's I had burned out my knees by teaching up to 5 aerobic classes per day (in my 20's), running long distances and cycling long distance. I stopped exercising altogether and gained over 60 lbs. I was so fed up with exercise that I did very little and spent more time recipe testing and wine tasting for my cookbooks. Now in my 50's I've finally learned the magic of patience and discipline as it relates to my health and weight. I eat a healthy, Gluten-Free diet, walk only 3 miles on a regular basis and drink wine moderately. I sample my recipes (instead of devouring the dishes) and I assess wines on a regular basis. I don't overindulge. My cholesterol is normal. I have low blood pressure and take no medications whatsoever.

This diet is about reaching a weight for overall health and to prevent and/or control diseases and conditions. When overweight, we put ourselves at risk of developing serious health issues, including heart disease, high blood pressure, type 2 diabetes, gallstones, breathing problems, cancers, sleep apnea, osteoarthritis, fatty liver disease, kidney disease, arthritis, to name but a few.

The Gluten-Free diet should be utilized to reach and maintain a healthy weight.

What is Gluten?
Gluten is a protein found in wheat, barley, and rye. It is a composite created when two proteins (glutenin and gliadin) are mixed with water and form hydrogen bonds, allowing them to form a sturdy network. It is this ability that has made gluten-containing grains preferable for baking bread and making pasta. Gluten creates structure. It allows bread to hold its shape, absorb moisture and become more elastic. It gives pasta that wonderful al dente texture. Gluten is readily used in soups, sauces, spices, gravies, and thickeners, and even in beer and liquor.

Oats are Gluten-Free, but can be gluten contaminated. Most commercial oats are processed in facilities that also process wheat, barley, and rye. So if you have Celiac disease or are highly sensitive to gluten, refrain from eating oats, unless you know they are free from contamination.

Any food that is but 1 ingredient cannot have gluten in it. Single ingredient products are good for us. Fruits, vegetables, meat, poultry and fish are healthy, as are lentils, nuts, corn, and rice. Even chocolate, wine and dairy products can be nutritional, when consumed in moderation.

2

There are distinctions to be made between Celiac disease, wheat allergies and gluten intolerance and sensitivity.

If you believe you may suffer from one of these conditions, it's extremely important to consult your doctor.

CHAPTER TWO: Health Concerns Related to Gluten

Even if you do not suffer from Celiac disease or gluten intolerance or sensitivity, the elimination of wheat, rye and barley can be beneficial to your health and help you lose weight. But let's look at this issue, first.

Celiac Disease and Diagnosis

Celiac disease is a lifelong autoimmune response caused by intolerance to gluten. It is life threatening. It is believed that 1 in every 100 people have this condition. There are no typical signs and symptoms of Celiac disease. However, symptoms include bloating, diarrhea, nausea, gas, constipation, tiredness, headaches, muscle cramps, sudden weight loss, hair loss, anemia, osteoporosis, and abdominal pain.

Sometimes people with Celiac disease have no abdominal symptoms at all. Instead, a person can suffer irritability, joint pain, muscle cramps, mouth sores, tingling in the feet, or a rash called Dermatitis herpetiformis – an itchy, blistering skin disease. It is estimated that about 10 percent of patients with Celiac disease also have this skin disorder.

A blood test showing elevated level of antibodies is an indication of Celiac disease. This indicates that one's immune system recognizes gluten as a foreign substance and increases the number of antibodies to fight it.

After the blood tests, the doctor will perform intestinal tissue to check for damage to the villi.

A thin, flexible tube is inserted through the mouth, esophagus and stomach and into the small intestine. The doctor then takes a small tissue sample. The tiny, hair-like projections from the small intestine that absorb vitamins, minerals and other nutrients will provide the necessary information.

After undergoing medical examination, a Gluten-Free trial period can confirm the diagnosis. It's important that the medical examination is done first. Otherwise, the diet may have an impact on the results of the blood test and biopsies. They may appear normal and without any complications even if the patient is positive with Celiac disease.

Wheat Allergy

Wheat allergies are also an immune response to wheat and to gluten. It is one of the most common allergies in children. It is often confused with Celiac disease or gluten sensitivity. A wheat allergy shows difference symptoms. Symptoms include swelling, itching or irritations of the mouth or throat, hives, rashes of the skin, nasal congestion, itchy and watery eyes, difficulty breathing, cramps, nausea or vomiting, diarrhea and anaphylaxis (tightening of the throat, fast heart beat, difficulty breathing, trouble swallowing, dizziness or fainting).

Gluten Sensitivity/Intolerance

Gluten intolerance and gluten sensitivity are terms highly disputed and difficult to distinguish, as opinions between scientists and physicians differ.

What we know is that it includes a spectrum of symptoms, disorders and effects. Those of us who suffer from gluten intolerance or sensitivity experience issues, such as bloating, abdominal pain, diarrhea, constipation, irritable bowel syndrome, muscular disturbances, headaches, migraines, acne, fatigue, bone and joint pain.

Check with Your Doctor

How many symptoms of gluten sensitivity or gluten intolerance might you have?

Digestive Issues:

Do you have frequent bloating or gas, irritable bowel syndrome or acid reflux? Do you suffer from daily diarrhea or chronic constipation?

Neurologic and Skeletal Issues:

Do you get migraines or headaches? Do you experience joint aches and pains? Does your mind occur as foggy?

Hormonal and Immune Issues:

Do you experience depression or anxiety? Are you always tired? Do you have eczema or acne?

If you experience even one of these symptoms, it's important to consult your doctor or try going Gluten-Free for 4 weeks. Or both.

The best test is to determine how you feel. It is best to listen to your own body by assessing how you feel after eating certain foods. Take note of how your body responds to different types of grain. Removing gluten-based grains from your diet can bring relief from digestive issues, skin rashes, joint pain, chronic fatigue, and even anxiety.

Everybody Else; With or Without Celiac or an Intolerance to Gluten

A Gluten-Free diet can be healthy and beneficial even if you are free from Celiac disease or gluten-intolerance or sensitivity.

Did you know that the average person consumes about 55 pounds of wheat products each year?

Wheat, alone, is grown on more land area around the planet than any other commercial food. The world trade in wheat is greater than for all other crops combined.

More and more physicians like Dr. Davis (author of the best selling book called Wheat Belly), neurologists like Dr. David Perlmutter (author of the best selling book called Grain Brain) and naturopathic doctors, such as Peter Glidden (advocate and speaker) believe that a wheat, rye and barley-free diet is a healthy lifestyle choice for everyone. It can help us heal our body, mind, and spirit and help us shed weight.

Dr. Glidden advocates that gluten is a difficult protein for the body to digest. Difficult for every human body. The reason is that protein (despite its source) has long chains of amino acids that are linked together through chemical bonds. There are 12 amino acids, which are essential nutrients that our body needs to import on a daily basis.

Our stomach is supposed to break the chemical bonds, liberating the free amino acids to be chewed and digested and absorbed. The source of the protein distinguishes its structure. The structure of protein can be vastly different from one source or ingredient to another. Herein lies the issue. The chemical bond in wheat, barley, and rye is difficult for the human stomach to digest.

It is through the small intestines that all the nutrition from food is absorbed. Our small intestines contain millions of villi. On top of the villi are thousands of microvilli. In our intestinal tract there are billions of tissues designed to absorb nutrients. It's the job of the villi to stick onto a molecule of digested food and suck the nutrients from it and put it into the blood stream. The body cannot utilize nutrients until they are digested and absorbed by the bloodstream.

The chemical bonds of wheat, barley, and rye are difficult to break. When the majority of people eat these products, the protein is left undigested. An undigested protein tumbling through the intestinal tract acts like a live wire, zapping and destroying the villi. It is the job of the villi to absorb nutrients. So if the villi are destroyed, the body is unable to absorb nutrients. The result is mal-absorption, which is the primary cause of most chronic diseases.

Be Careful; Be Smart

If you are suffering from major symptoms like irritable bowel syndrome or inflammatory bowel disease, do not assume that going Gluten-Free will cure these issues and symptoms. Irritable bowel syndrome (IBS) and inflammatory bowel disease and lactose intolerance can be symptoms of gluten-intolerance. But they can also be symptoms of other serious issues at work, as well. Irritable bowel syndrome is a gastrointestinal (GI) disorder caused by changes in the GI tract. The causes of IBS are still not well understood. It is believed that a brain-gut signal issue, a GI motor issue, hypersensitivity, mental health issues, bacterial gastroenteritis, and small intestinal bacterial overgrowth, genetics and body chemicals can cause it. Removing gluten from your diet may cause health problems by restricting your intake of important vitamins and minerals. So if you suffer from serious symptoms, be sure to consult your doctor before starting a Gluten-Free diet.

CHAPTER THREE: Super Glutens and Frankenwheat

What's important to know is that the wheat we consume today and the super rate in which we incorporate wheat into our diet through a plethora of products is not the same wheat consumed by our ancestors. Today's wheat is considered by many to be a Frankenstein version of the original grain.

There are 3 cultivated wheat species. They are Diplois, Diploid and Tetrapoid. Wheat varieties within each species have varying levels of the gluten proteins called gliadin and glutenin. Gliadin is the soluble element in gluten; glutenin is the insoluble one.

Those suffering from Celiac disease or gluten-intolerance are reacting to gliadin protein. Gliadin causes an inflammatory reaction as it comes into contact with the wall of the small intestine. This low-grade inflammation may go undetected for years before symptoms become obvious. This can cause a slow destruction of the healthy living tissues within the small intestine. Over time gliadin intolerance creates significant stress on the immune system.

Our ancestors were found in the Great Rift Valley of Africa about 2.6 million years ago, which ended about 15,000 BC. During this era our ancestors consumed a wild species of wheat called Einkorn. Einkorn (of the Diplois species) is non-genetically altered with 14 chromosomes of gliadin.

In the 1950's scientists began crossbreeding and hybridizing wheat to make it hardier, shorter, and able to resist pests and diseases. As crop rotation was applied to long cultivated land, along with the use of fertilizers, yields of wheat increased. Wheat was required to feed larger populations of people across the globe. What we now know is that this morphing of wheat from its ancient form to its present version also introduced compounds believed to be unfriendly to the human digestive system.

Today's wheat variety (called bread or common wheat) and part of the Diploid species, is the most widely grown and used for the production of almost all commercial wheat products today. Common wheat has strong and elastic gluten that enables its dough to trap carbon dioxide during leavening and is therefore beneficial in the making of baked products like bread. The issue is that common wheat has a grand total of 42 chromosomes of gliadin -- not 14 like its ancestral version.

Durum wheat (part of the Tetrapoid species) is used for making pasta and contains 28 chromosomes of gliadin.

Durum and Bread wheat contain more than double and triple the amount of the protein gliadin as found in the ancient grain Einkorn. These hybridized and crossbred varieties are often referred to as 'super glutens' or 'Frankenwheats.'

Why should we care about the level of the protein gliadin in our breads and pastas? The reason is that high levels of gliadin are believed to trigger inflammation in the body. Inflammation then triggers insulin resistance, causing an increase in the appetite, gradual weight gain, and ultimately diabetes.

Research shows that super gluten wheat raises blood sugar levels, causing immunoreactive problems, inhibits the absorption of important minerals, and aggravates our intestines. These wheat are now believed by many scientists and experts to contribute to obesity, diabetes, heart disease, cancer, dementia, depression and a plethora of other illnesses.

(Keep in mind that there are researchers, scientists, physicians and experts on the other side of the argument who will adamantly argue that wheat does not lead to these health conditions. They believe that if you are not suffering from Celiac disease or gluten sensitivity, then removing it from the diet is unnecessary and even ludicrous.)

No source of Frankenwheat — not newly sprouted or in baked bread, pasta or pastries -- is good for us.

Other Grains with Gliadin Structures

Rye and barley share similar gliadin structures to wheat.

There is much controversy over corn. In relation to Celiac disease, corn has not been studied to the same extent as wheat. But thus far, studies show that corn proteins on the celiac intestine are safe.

CHAPTER FOUR: The Gluten-Free Diet

Processed Gluten-Free Foods

According to a study by researchers at Dalhousie University in Halifax, Canada, published in the Canadian Journal of Dietetic Practice and Research in 2008, Gluten-Free products are a $4.2 billion dollar enterprise in the United States; $90-million in Canada.

This study also revealed that Gluten-Free products are 242% more expensive than their regular counterparts, and 455% pricier in some cases.

This is certainly true for me. I pay over $6.00 for a loaf of frozen Gluten-Free bread, but I eat so little of it, that it's worth the investment.

Gluten-Free packaged food is a huge market. They are convenient, but many have more sugar, fat and calories added. Or the fiber has been removed. There is no need to go this route.

"Being Gluten-Free is a good thing, but eating Gluten-Free processed foods is not a good thing," says Dr. William Davis, author of the best-selling book Wheat Belly: Lose the Wheat, Lose the Weight and Find Your Path Back to Health and US cardiologist. (CTVNews.ca)

Eating too much Gluten-Free processed food (what I call Gluten-Free junk food) like Gluten-Free cookies, cakes and processed food has a high glycemic load on your system. Just because it is Gluten-Free, doesn't mean it is healthy. Gluten-Free cakes and cookies are still cakes and cookies! Vegetables, fruits, beans, nuts and seeds and lean animal protein are all Gluten-Free -- stick with those.

"We don't want to replace one problem with other problems," says Dr. Davis. "Foods that raise your blood sugar sky-high, make your tummy grow, give you hyper-tension, dementia, cancer and heart disease." (CTVNews.ca)

The Benefits of Going Gluten-Free

Dr. William Davis wrote an extraordinary article in Life Extension Magazine, Oct. 2011. It is called Wheat: The Unhealthy Whole Grain Book Excerpt: Wheat Belly. It is worth reading, as it explains from a scientific perspective the issues related to wheat consumption and its impact on the body.

Weight Loss

The Gluten-Free diet supports the notion of eating single ingredient foods – fruits, vegetables, fish, poultry and lean meats. It embodies the philosophy of staying away from Gluten-Free boxed and processed foods that are usually high in calories, sugar, fat and preservatives. It means focusing on and eating low glycemic Gluten-Free grains that do not stimulate the appetite or raise your blood sugar levels. And it means consuming products, such as dairy, chocolate and wine in moderation. These elements ultimately lead to gradual weight loss over time. Going Gluten-Free is by no means a crash diet.

Improved Digestion

The second benefit of a Gluten-Free Diet is that it greatly maintains and improves the digestive system. A lot of people who have gone on a Gluten-Free diet noticed a mild to drastic change in terms of their digestion in a short period of time. They have said that there has been a noticeable improvement in bowel movements and a great reduction in indigestion. There is also a significant decrease in bloating and cramps, which is a definite plus for women.

Reduced Joint Inflammation

The third benefit of a Gluten-Free Diet is that it reduces inflammation in various tissues in the body. People who are highly sensitive and allergic to gluten usually experience episodes of pain in joints, muscles, and legs. People who also experience inflammation on the skin such as Dermatitis, Eczema, or Dermatitis Herpetiformis will reap some benefits from a Gluten-Free diet, as well.

My husband has noticed that he experiences less pain in his hips and knees.

Increased Energy Levels

The fourth benefit of a Gluten-Free Diet is that it improves energy levels especially in those people who suffer from Celiac disease, sensitivity or intolerance to gluten. It has been reported that people who consume too much gluten experience a lot of tiredness and weakness. Gluten-related fatigue can be disruptive and even debilitating.

Researches are still not entirely clear what causes fatigue in those with Celiac disease or gluten-intolerance. But fatigue is recognized as one of the top symptoms. One speculation is that fatigue is caused by malnutrition or anemia.

You may find that you also require more sleep than others.

While still not scientifically proven, gluten ingestion plays a direct role in sleep problems for people with Celiac disease and gluten sensitivity. Dr. Rodney Ford, a New Zealand pediatrician and author of *The Gluten Syndrome*, believes that a gluten diet affects the brain and neurological tissue directly. This causes symptoms. However, there is no direct research revealing this fact.

Reducing one's gluten intake or simply going Gluten-Free will help to support you getting those energy levels pumping.

Improved Blood-Sugar Levels

The fifth benefit is that going Gluten-Free will help keep your blood sugar levels at bay. A lot of food products that have gluten in them are usually accompanied by a significant amount of sugar. So switching to a diet made up of the consumption of more single ingredients like fruits and vegetables, foods that do not contain gluten, will help you to control your blood sugar and fat intake.

CHAPTER FIVE: What Kind of Taster Are You?

Other contributing factors can support you in reaching and maintaining your ideal weight. Have you ever found yourself, after eating a full course meal, gazing through the refrigerator knowing you wanted to something to eat and also knowing you were not very hungry? You close the refrigerator, only to find yourself opening it again in an hour or so.

This apparent phenomenon has to do with your palate being left unsatisfied even though your stomach may be full.

There's an old adage that says that some eat to live while others live to eat. It all has to do with the amount of taste buds we have, which ultimately affects our health and our weight! Yes, our taste buds affect our weight.

Dr. Bartoshuk is an internationally renowned researcher, now at the University of Florida, who specializes in the chemical senses of taste and smell. She has conducted research into genetic variations in taste perception, oral pain and taste disorders.

According to Dr. Bartoshuk, taste buds are sensory organs on the tongue that allow us to experience tastes. Our sensory sensations differ according to the number and distribution of our taste buds.

Everyone produces a varying amount of saliva, and at a different rate, which also affects perception of taste.

Dr. Bartoshuk says people are born with a genetically determined number of taste buds and divides them into three groups, according to the number of taste buds they have. Super-tasters account for about 25% of the population, tasters about 50% and non-tasters at 25%. It is the non-tasters who are more likely to gain weight.

According to Dr. Bartoshuk, super-tasters possess more taste buds than medium or non-tasters. As a result, they experience the taste, temperature and texture of foods, most specifically bitterness, more keenly than tasters or non-tasters. Super-tasters tend to avoid green vegetables because they taste too bitter or sharp. Coffee and scotch are also bitter tasting to the super-taster. They tend to avoid high-fat foods, sweets, and fruits and vegetables because the flavors are too intense. To the super-taster, espresso, olives, arugula, dark chocolate and dry wines can taste too bitter and are therefore not palatable. Super-tasters experience intense tastes and oral burns from chemical irritants such as chili peppers, black pepper and cayenne. Super tasters tend to be lean.

Those with a less acute sense of taste are called non-tasters (such as myself) are more likely to gain weight. We cannot discern the taste of fat, which explains why we crave higher-fat foods. We also crave sweet and salty foods. Our sense of taste influences our food choices that ultimately determine our weight.

Non-tasters require an over load of flavor to experience satisfaction. I enjoy stinky blue cheese over mozzarella and black coffee over double double. For me scotch tastes sweet. To experience meal satisfaction, my food must be heavily seasoned and spiced. I devour Indian and Thai curries. Research is now showing that non-tasters are experiencing more heart and stroke related diseases due to our being overweight and consuming fatty foods. Our preference for high seasonings, sweet and fatty foods means most of us are overweight.

The medium taster can fluctuate to either side of this scale. The kind of taster we are also contributes to the state of our health and, again, our weight.

As a non-taster, I assault and no doubt damage my tongue by regularly consuming lots of hot sauce and raw garlic. Fortunately, the taste system is built with a lot of redundancy, so even when parts of it are damaged, whole mouth taste stays relatively constant.

In your quest to lose weight on your Gluten-Free diet, it's also important to understand the kind of taster you are. Said another way this knowledge will allow you to become more conscious of why you choose the foods you choose. This knowledge can help loosen the grip that the food addiction hand has around our throats!

Are you a super-taster, medium-taster or non- taster? Why not test yourself? You'll need a cotton swab, polyvinyl ring (used for reinforcing punched holes in binder paper), blue food coloring, a mirror and a magnifying glass. Place the ring on your tongue near the front, not on the tip. Using the cotton swab put a tiny drop of food coloring inside the ring.

Use the mirror to look at your tongue through the magnifying glass. Pink dots will emerge through the blue dye. The dots are fungiform papillae, mushroom-shaped structures containing taste buds. If you have more than 35 dots in that area, you're a super-taster. If you have 15 to 35, you're a medium-taster. Fewer than 10 make you a non-taster.

There's another factor at work with respect to our sense of taste and our weight and it tends to affect non-tasters the most. If we eat processed foods from the grocery store or even fast food chain, we numb our taste buds. Our taste buds become confused by the layering of conflicting flavors, such as too much saltiness, upon sweetness (sugar), upon fattiness. This forces our taste buds into overdrive. As a result our taste buds lose their sensitivity. This has us eat more food in hopes of satisfying our taste buds. (Super tasters tend to eat less.)

But don't get discouraged. You can recalibrate your taste buds. Simply cut back on all processed foods for a few weeks or longer. Stay away from fast food chain restaurants, cut back on fat and try not to add additional salt. Just for a few weeks until your palate is recalibrated.

17

If you're a non-taster like me once recalibrated choose foods that are low in calories and fat and high in spice. This will help you lose those extra pounds all the while satisfying your palate. Try Kimchi. I love it and it's exactly what I need. It's Gluten-Free.

Kimchi is a spicy Korean, fermented cabbage dish packed with nutrition. It is made with cut cabbage, radish, and scallions and a seasoned paste of Korean red pepper, garlic, fresh ginger, sugar, and fish sauce, salted shrimp, or kelp powder.

It can be eaten alone or included in salads, sandwiches, stir-fries and soups. And 2/3 cup serving has only about 40 calories. According to medical reports, this delicacy is also packed with various probiotics that help to balance the bacterial environment in the digestive system. It is low in cholesterol, fat, and carbohydrates and is packed with antioxidants, vitamins A and C.

Keep in mind that you should not be eating kimchi if you are re-calibrating your palate or suffer from cardiovascular disease. It is high in sodium. It should also be eaten in moderation because it does contain low levels of carcinogen. **(Kimchi contains N-nitroso compounds, which are likely carcinogens.)** While classic Kimchi calls for sugar, you can use Asian pear as a substitute.

Here is a recipe:

Kimchi
1 large (5 pound) Napa cabbage
1/2 cup coarse salt
1/4 cup sweet rice flour (mochi)*
1 cup water
1/2 cup Gluten-free fish sauce or Gluten-Free soy sauce for a vegetarian version
2 cups Korean red chili flakes*
1/2 cup garlic, chopped
1 tbsp. ginger, grated
1 small onion, grated

18

1/2 Asian pear, grated
1/2 Fuji apple, grated
1 cup daikon radish shredded*
1/4 cup carrot, shredded
1 bunch green onions, sliced

*Can be purchased at Asian supermarkets
Cut the Napa cabbage in half, remove the core and slice the cabbage into 1-inch wide strips. Soak the cabbage in cold water for 10 minutes.

Place a layer of cabbage into a large bowl and sprinkle some salt onto the cabbage. Repeat until all of the cabbage is in the bowl and salted. (Use two bowls if needed.) Let the cabbage sit for 1 1/2 hours mixing it up every 1/2 hour. Rinse the cabbage three times, drain and set aside.

Mix the flour and water in a small saucepan and bring to a simmer while stirring. Remove from heat and let it cool. Mix flour mixture and the remaining ingredients, save the cabbage. Mix the porridge into the cabbage well using your hands to make sure that it covers all of the cabbage. Place the cabbage mixture into sealable containers leaving about an inch of space at the top. Seal the container and let ferment at room temperature for 2-3 days. Place the container in the fridge and let ferment for a couple more days.

CHAPTER SIX: A Family Approach

A family that eats together heals together.

On a Gluten-Free diet, you'll need to think about what foods to buy, grow, store, prepare or eat at any time of the day. It is not just about ensuring that food is Gluten-Free but also ensuring that the essential nutrients are sourced from all food groups.

If you live in a family situation, this will require some planning. You can also seek help from a dietician for the information on Gluten-Free foods. A dietitian can help you and your family learn how to read labels that may not specify gluten but contain it nonetheless. An example is an ingredient called hydrolyzed vegetable protein doesn't tell you that it has been sourced from wheat.

It is not just about knowing what to avoid, but rather knowing what to eat. For example, fruits are very much encouraged to reduce other stressors to the digestive system, such as constipation. Further, in planning what meals to prepare and what other food to stock in the kitchen, you and your family can treat this as an opportunity to monitor and ensure balanced nutrition and sufficient caloric intake.

But what happens when family members, especially the children, need to eat outside of the home?

Again, it is important for the family to plan ahead. Children and teens should be part of the whole process of learning about Gluten-Free food.

To engage their interest and to ensure that they like what they eat, children and teens may be entrusted with the responsibility of choosing what Gluten-Free meals to prepare. In this way, they would be able to prepare for food they can either eat at home or have as packed lunch or snacks. But in cases when they have to buy food outside the home, their knowledge about Gluten-Free food would enable them to discriminate which meals to buy. For young children with Celiac disease, their parents can also talk to teachers about the food requirements of their children. Or talk to the parents of their children's friends, in case they visit or sleep over at houses of their friends.

CHAPTER SEVEN: Gluten-Free Grains that Support Weight Loss

A study published in the *American Journal of Clinical Nutrition* underscores the importance of choosing whole grains such as brown rice rather than refined grain, i.e., white rice, to maintain a healthy body weight. In this Harvard Medical School / Brigham and Women's Hospital study, which collected data on over 74,000 female nurses aged 38-63 years over a 12 year period, weight gain was associated with the intake of refined-grain foods. It revealed that women who consumed more whole grains were 49% less likely to gain weight compared to those eating foods made from refined grains.

The Gluten-Free diet requires the complete elimination of all wheat, rye and barley products.

Gluten-Free replacements for cereals and baking mixes are often made up of a combination of cornstarch, potato starch, tapioca starch and/or white rice flour. The nutrient composition of these ingredients falls short in comparison to those provided by whole grains.

That's why it is important for you incorporate Gluten-Free whole grains into your diet on a daily basis. Without whole grains, you can become deficient in important minerals, vitamins, fiber, calcium, and iron.

Store whole grains in airtight containers. Store them for no longer than a year in a cool, dark place. Millet should be consumed within 2 to 3 months. Whole grain flours will last up to 6 months or in the freezer for up to a year.

When cooking whole grains, remember that they double or triple in size once cooked. For flavoring add broths, stocks, juice or milk in place of water. Before cooking grains, be sure to rinse them first. Bring the liquid to a boil and then reduce to simmer. You need not stir the grains. Once the grains absorb the liquid and are tender, remove them from the heat and let them sit for about 5 minutes.

Cook more than you need and store the extra cooked grains in the freezer.

On the Gluten-Free diet, there are whole grains that support weight loss and others that sabotage it.

Despite its name, buckwheat is not wheat. In fact, it isn't a grain at all. It's a fruit seed of a plant that is related to rhubarb. These grain-like seeds have a unique triangular shape and are the same size as wheat kernels. Buckwheat can be ground into flour and substitute wheat, rye, barley and oats in recipes.

If you are embracing the Gluten-Free diet, then you'll want to also embrace this fruit! It is fat free, low in calories, fills you up faster, controls blood sugar, facilitates proper digestion, builds lean muscle mass and suppresses the appetite. What more can you ask for in a seed?

Buckwheat

Buckwheat contains a medicinal chemical that strengthens capillary walls and reduces hemorrhage, thus lowering the risk of fatal strokes and heart attacks in people with high blood pressure and diabetes. It improves micro vascular integrity and circulation in diabetics, thus preventing the damage of nerves and muscle cells and loss of kidney function.

As a good source of magnesium, Buckwheat helps to improve blood pressure by relaxing the blood vessels. As a rich source of B vitamins (niacin, folate and B6), this seed contributes toward our cardiovascular health. These vitamins reduce the concentration of cholesterol in the blood and increases in high-density lipoproteins (HDL). This further enhances blood vessel strength and bad cholesterol removal. Buckwheat's iron, magnesium, phosphorus, copper and manganese help in reduce blood pressure and improve blood oxygenation. It contains high quality proteins (containing all 8 essential amino acids), which remove the plaque forming triglycerides and low-density lipoproteins (LDL). Thus buckwheat is highly beneficial for all of us, especially those with weak heart functions and other cardiovascular problems.

Buckwheat contains D-chiro-Inositol. This is a compound that is deficient in type II diabetic patients and is required for proper conduction of insulin for controlling and treating type II diabetes.

Because it is composed of cellulose, buckwheat removes toxins from the body, acting as a cleansing ingredient. And as an insoluble fiber, Buckwheat helps to prevent gallstones. It speeds up the removal of food through the intestines, increases insulin sensitivity but lowers the secretion of bile acids and blood sugar.

A diet rich in Buckwheat can also help reduce the risk of breast cancer. Its antioxidant properties are also beneficial for women during and after menopause, thus protecting against the risk of breast cancer and other forms of cancers related to hormones.

Buckwheat has a plethora of other health benefits, as well. It strengthens bones by facilitating the absorption of calcium. It contains tryptophan to influence our mood and helps to prevent depression and strengthens our immune system against flu and the common cold.

The key to implementing buckwheat for weight loss is to eat it partially raw. When it is cooked buckwheat loses its nutrients and properties and its abilities to clean the body. When toasted, buckwheat is called Kasha. In Russia, Kasha is served with onions and brown gravy.

To Cook: There is a sweet spot for where your buckwheat will be tender enough to eat, but not mushy. Bring 2 cups of water to a boil in a medium saucepan with some salt. Stir in 1 cup of buckwheat and bring back to a boil. Keep the lid off. Once the buckwheat starts to expand and all the visible water is absorbed, turn down the heat to low and place the lid on the pot.

Leave the buckwheat to cook for another 5 to 15 minutes, depending on the consistency you desire. Check it regularly.

Quinoa

Quinoa originated in South America and has been a staple in the South American diet for centuries. More than a grain it is a seed relative of spinach, kale and Swiss chard. As a super food, it is low in calories and rich in dietary fiber and protein and low in calories.

Quinoa is also low on the glycemic index, as low as vegetables. (The glycemic index indicates how carbohydrates affect your blood glucose.) It won't spike your blood sugar. When your blood sugar is unbalanced, staying on a diet and making healthy eating choices is difficult because of cravings for sweets and refined breads.

Due to its fiber content, quinoa makes you feel full much faster. Its dietary fiber binds to fat and cholesterol, which causes your body to absorb less fat and cholesterol. The fiber found in quinoa also reduces the plaque build-up along your arterial walls, which reduces your risk of heart disease and stroke. Quinoa contains high quality protein and has a protein profile similar to cow's milk. It is an excellent source of iron, calcium, magnesium, B Vitamins and riboflavin.

(Be sure to rinse it several times before cooking to remove the bitter coating.)

To Cook: Rinse it well. There is a bitter coating on the tiny seed that needs to be rinsed away. When rinsing it, use a fine-mesh strainer. Combine 1 cup of quinoa with 2 cups of water in a medium saucepan. Bring to a boil. Cover, reduce heat to low and simmer until quinoa is tender, about 15 minutes. When cooked, drain the quinoa for 15 minutes; otherwise your dish will be watery. Return quinoa to the hot pot. This allows it to dry out.

Brown Rice

Because of its high fiber content, brown rice fills the stomach more quickly. This general leads to automatic smaller meal portions, thus inadvertently helping you eat less.

While requiring a long cooking time, brown rice is considered one of the world's healthiest foods. It is the whole grain with its inedible outer hull removed, while still retaining its nutrient-rich bran and germ. (White rice is both milled and polished, removing the bran and germ along with all the other layer-rich nutrients).

Some of the most popular varieties include: Long grain brown rice, with springy character, is well suited for casseroles and baked dishes. Medium grain brown rice is stickier and ideal for Spanish dishes like paellas. Short grain brown rice has creamy texture and can be used in risotto. Brown basmati rice is firm and has a dry consistency, ideal for biryanis and pilafs. Aromatic jasmine rice is moist and tender and good for Asian dishes and Kalijira rice grains are fast cooking and can substitute couscous-based dishes

One cup of brown rice provides your body with 80% of its daily manganese requirement. Manganese is important to help your body synthesize fats. Brown rice comes in short, medium and long lengths and in a whole bunch of different varieties with flavors and aromas. It is a good source of selenium, phosphorus, copper, magnesium, and niacin and fiber, fatty acids, amino acids and more. Due to its massive nutritional value, brown rice supports the prevention of ailments, including heart disease, cancers, diabetes, gallstones, decreasing asthma and the inflammation of rheumatoid arthritis.

To Cook: Rinse rice until the water runs clear. In a medium saucepan add 2 tablespoons of olive oil. Heat the oil, then add 1 cup of rice. This helps to build the flavor of the rice. Add 2.5 cups of water and a pinch of salt and bring to a boil. Reduce the heat to simmer, cover the pot and let simmer until the rice is tender, about 40 minutes. When the rice has finished cooking and the water has boiled off, let it rest with the lid on, for about 5 minutes.

Teff

Teff has been a staple in the Ethiopian diet for thousands of years. It is an ancient North African cereal grass and a super food! The germ and bran, where the nutrients are concentrated, account for a larger volume of the seed compared to the more popular grains. It is also the world's smallest grain and is 40% resistant starch, meaning that half the calories consumed cannot be absorbed.

Resistant starch foods like teff can help you lose weight if you use it as a substitute for pasta. What's unique about Teff is packed with Vitamin C. Grains are normally devoid of this vitamin. Teff possess the eight essential amino acids a body needs in order to properly grow. Teff also helps manage the body's blood sugar levels and triggers bowel movement to perform properly.

It has a mild, nutty flavor and can be used to make polenta, cookies, breads, stews and so much more.

To Cook: Rinse teff under cold water. Add 1 cup of rinsed teff and 3 cups of water to a pot. Bring to a boil. Turn the heat to simmer, cover the pot and let cook for about 10 to 15 minutes. Turn off the heat, and let the teff sit for about 10 minutes. This allows the teff to absorb all the water. It should be sticky and nutty.

Amaranth

Considered a weed by much of the world, Amaranth was used by the Aztecs as a food staple. It is not really a grain, but rather a seed belonging to the Amaranthaceae family. This seed has a significant amount of the essential vitamins A, C, E, K, B5, B6, folate, niacin and riboflavin. These act as antioxidants, increase energy and control hormones. It is also rich in lysine (an amino acid) calcium, potassium, iron, copper, magnesium, phosphorus and manganese, protein, dietary fiber, and amino acids — all essential for a healthy body. Amino acids, lysine in particular, are said to reduce the risk of cancer and lowers bad cholesterol. Amaranth is also great in boosting the immune system. It helps fight off certain diseases such as cardiovascular and hypertension.

Amaranth's moderately high content of oxalic acid inhibits much of the absorption of calcium and zinc. It should be avoided or eaten in moderation by those inflicted with gout, kidney disorders or rheumatoid arthritis.

To Cook: 1 cup of amaranth to 3 cups of water. Bring to a boil, and then simmer for 25 minutes. The final consistency will be thick, like porridge. If you want to combine amaranth with another grain, substitute it with about ¼ of the other grain, then cook as you would for that grain.

Sorghum

Originating in Africa about 8000 years ago, Sorghum is a cereal grain used in Gluten-Free cooking. Because it doesn't possess an inedible hull like other grains, Sorghum is commonly eaten with all its outer layers, thereby providing your body with its nutrients. It is also grown from traditional hybrid seeds and so does not contain traits gained through biotechnology. It is non-transgenic (non-GMO). It is great for weight loss as Sorghum digests more slowly with a lower glycemic index, and so sticks with you a bit longer than other flours or flour substitutes. It also helps to speed up the metabolism and at the same time supports it. Sorghum contains a lot of magnesium and copper, minerals playing an important role in proper food metabolizing. Packed with antioxidants, this cereal helps to reduce the risk of cancer development and cardiovascular disease.

Sorghum can be substituted for wheat flour in a variety of recipes. It's neutral, sometimes sweet and is easily adaptable. It improves the texture of recipes.

To Cook: Rinse, drain and pick through sorghum. Combine 3 cups of water or stock with 1 cup of Sorghum in a pot with a lid.

Bring to a boil. Cover, reduce the heat to low and let simmer for about 50 to 60 minutes. Drain any excess water.

Gluten-Free Grains that Support Weight Gain

Millet

Originating in China, this particular grain can be used as a substitute for rice-based recipes; even risotto or polenta as it develops a creamy based texture.

It is high in B vitamins and fiber and is provides alkalizing benefits to the body. In terms of taste, Millet has a sugary yet nutty flavor. This particular grain is digestible and only a few people are known to be allergic to it. Millet also prevents constipation by making sure the colon is well hydrated. Millet is considered as a smart carb, since it contains an immense amount of fiber and low plain sugars, which helps in keeping the blood sugar levels of the body healthy and in tip-top shape.

BUT, do not over indulge in eating millet if you want to lose weight. Millet contains goitrogen, which increases after cooking. Goitrogen is believed to suppress thyroid activity and can lead to depression, difficulty in losing weight, and fatigue.

Whole Grain Cornmeal

While whole grain cornmeal contains a lot of vitamins and minerals such as iron, phosphorus, magnesium, zinc, and vitamin B-6, it is also high in calories. So eat it sparingly if you want to lose weight through the Gluten-Free diet. One cup of cornmeal has 500 calories! According to research, cornmeal is said to be great in helping improve digestion, reduce high blood pressure, and lessen the risk of acquiring heart disease, gallstones, etc.

CHAPTER EIGHT: Starch Can Be a Good Thing

Resistant starch is getting more attention of late as they have received praise from the Food and Agricultural Organization (FAO) and World Health Organization (WHO). In fact there have been hundreds of studies revealing that resistant starch is a healthy food group for weight loss and management, glycemic control and digestive health.

Simply put, resistant starch is a type of starch that moves completely through the small intestine without being digested. As a result these starches resist digestion and act like soluble fiber. They help to lower fat levels because they have less energy and consequently fewer calories than other starches. They assist the fermentation of good bacteria that can affect our hormones, body fat, and glucose and glycemic index levels in a way that encourages weight loss.

Research has shown that resistant starch foods have health benefits, such as:

Promotes satiation to encourage weight loss
Decreases hunger to encourage weight loss
Affects glycemic index levels to encourage weight loss
Positively affects our hormones
Improves insulin resistance
Lowers insulin and glucose levels after meals
Makes more butyrate than other prebiotics
Lowers the risk of bowel cancer
Bolsters immune system
Improves gastrointestinal health
Improves kidney health

Resistant starches take a considerably longer time to digest. That means expanding as they soak up fluids in your body stimulating satiety and giving you effective control over your appetite.

Here is a list of resistant starch foods to include in your Gluten-Free menu whenever possible:

Green Bananas (1 medium peeled, 4.7 g of resistant starch)

In North America we seem to only like to ripe bananas. But green bananas are an integral part of other cultural menus, such as in the Caribbean and Jamaica. Bananas contain inulin, a resistant starch that serves as a strong probiotic in the body, improving health gut flora as well as controlling blood sugar. I like to incorporate green bananas into bread. It's fabulous in shakes and frozen yogurt.

White Beans (1/2-cup, prepared, 4.5 g)

White beans offer a double benefit for the Gluten-Free dieter. They are high in resistant starch. They also are low in fat. Beans reduce blood sugar, and create the fatty acid butyrate, which burns fat faster. Studies have shown that butyrate improves mitochondrial function in your cells, leading to a decrease in fat. If you are concerned about gas, fret not. The more beans you eat, the more your body will build up the good bacteria to digest them. I love to puree white beans with garlic, fresh lemon juice, Parmigiano-Reggiano and salt and pepper to taste. Spread the mixture of toast. It is a tasty hors d'oeuvre. It can also be served as a dip.

Lentils (1/2-cup, 3.7 g)

Lentils are legumes, the seeds of plants whose botanical name is Lens Ensculenta. In North America we consume green or brown lentils. But they are also available in black, yellow, red and orange. Lentils readily absorb the flavors of the other ingredients in a dish and they have high nutritional value, as well as being a high resistant starch with no fat! Lentils are a good source of cholesterol lowering fiber and prevent the blood-sugar level from rising after a meal. While giving the body energy, lentils also can help reduce the risk of coronary heart disease and cardiovascular disease. They are a good source of folate, copper, phosphorus, manganese, iron, protein, B1, zinc, potassium and vitamin B6. Before cooking lentils spread them out and remove any stones. Then wash them thoroughly. Place them in boiling water for 20 to 30 minutes, depending on their end use. Often this legume gets over looked or type-casted in the roll as a soup and stew ingredient. But lentils can be used in making burgers, omelets, dips, chili, sloppy Joes, vegetarian Moussaka, tacos, Indian Mango Dal, risotto, salads and even cabbage rolls.

Yams (1/2-cup, cooked, 2.5 g)

I probably eat more sweet potato than yams. But yams are a resistant starch and certainly more enticing from this perspective. Yams are different than sweet potatoes. The flesh inside a sweet potato is orange. The flesh inside a yam is white to purple. Yam is the starchier and drier distant cousin of sweet potato. It originated in Africa where 95 percent of the crops are still grown. The rough scaly skin ranges from off-white to dark brown. Yams are low in fat and are a good source of vitamin C, B6, thiamin, manganese, copper and potassium. It is a healthy complex carbohydrate that helps the digestive tract and aids in decreasing the risk of obesity, heart disease and several forms of cancer.

We tend to stick to one yam dish – candied yams. But yams can be incorporated into the bean burrito, stews and soups, kebabs, breads, mashed with potatoes, garlic and Parmesan and more.

Chickpeas (1/2-cup, prepared, 2.0 g)

I think my husband and I survive on chickpea dip called hummus with Gluten-Free tortilla chips. It certainly wards off hunger pains until dinner. In a food processer or blender combine 2 cups of canned chickpeas (drained and rinsed) with 3 tablespoons of tahini, 2 cloves of garlic, 2 tablespoons of lemon juice, ¼ cup of coconut or olive oil, and kosher salt and black pepper to taste. This Middle Eastern legume can also be used in salads, burgers, and soups. Chickpeas can also be pureed with yogurt and cumin and served as a dip. Besides being a resistant starch, chickpeas boost your energy, stabilize blood sugar levels and are high in protein and have a low glycemic index. They reduce bad cholesterol, aiding in the reduction of the risk of heart disease.

Green peas (1/2-cup, prepared, 2.0 g)
Green peas are not as powerful a resistant starch as green bananas, but they are packed with other nutrition that's hard to beat.

Green peas, in the legume family, are a nutritionally loaded addition to soups, salads, as a side dish, or in stir-fries and noodle dishes, to name but a few. They contain important fat-soluble nutrients like beta-carotene, vitamin E, omega-6 fatty acid and linoleic acid. Some other green pea health benefits include anti-aging, a strong immune system and high energy. These benefits come from their flavonoids (catechin and epicatechin), carotenoid (alpha and beta-carotene), phenolic acids (ferulic and caffeic acids) and polyphenols (coumestrol).

Due to their strong anti-inflammatory properties, vitamins C and E and Omega-3 fat, this legume also helps to prevent wrinkles, Alzheimer's, arthritis, bronchitis, and candida. They are high in fiber and so regulate the blood sugar level, aid in the reversal of insulin resistance (type 2 diabetes) and improve bowel health. With an abundance of vitamin B1 and folate, B2, B3, and B6, vitamin K (anchors calcium), green peas aid in the prevention of heart disease and osteoporosis.

When purchasing fresh green peas look for pods that are firm and smooth. They should have a medium green color and flat. If the color is dark, yellow, whitish or specked with gray, avoid them.

Brown Rice (½ cup, cooked, 1.6 g)
Brown Rice is covered in Chapter 7.

Kidney Beans (1/2-cup, prepared, 1.4 g)
I've been studying the many benefits of beans, specifically kidney beans. When combined with rice, this legume provides an excellent source of protein – without the high calories and fat of red meat! In fact, one cup of kidney beans provides 15.3 grams of protein, 30% of one's daily requirement.

Like most beans, kidneys are also an excellent source of cholesterol lowering fiber. Hypoglycemic and diabetic friendly, these beans help to stabilize blood sugar levels after meals.

One of the best benefits of kidneys is that they are high in 'molybdenum.' Molybdenum is a trace mineral and an important part of the enzyme sulfite oxidase, which is responsible for detoxifying sulfites in the body.

One cup of cooked kidney beans supplies about 177.0% of our molybdenum daily requirement. I checked my multivitamin. It contains 8 mcg of this trace mineral. For the human being, 75 mcg of molybdenum is a daily requirement. So, kidney beans are now a part of my weekly repertoire.

Molybdenum is believed to help to protect the stomach and esophagus against cancers, aids in the absorption of iron and so helps to prevent anemia, as well as tooth decay. Molybdenum also aids in the metabolizing of fats and carbohydrates. (Other than kidney beans, other foods high in molybdenum are meats, buckwheat, barley, wheat germ, lima beans, sunflower seeds and dark green leafy vegetables.)

Most importantly, kidney beans are high in soluble and insoluble fiber. Soluble fiber produces a gel-like substance that increases stool bulk and therefore helps to prevent constipation.

When buying kidney beans at bulk food stores, look closely to ensure they are not cracked, thus indicating too much moisture content.

To prepare dried kidneys quickly and for culinary greatness, rinse the beans under cool water. Place them in a pot on a burner with just enough water to cover. Bring the water to a boil and then let the beans simmer for 2 minutes. Remove the pan from the heat. Let the beans stand in their liquid for two hours. Remove the beans from this liquid. Discard the liquid. Rinse the beans under cool water again. Put them into a clean pot. Add 3 cups of water to every 1 cup of beans. Bring the water to a boil. Reduce the heat to simmer. Let the kidneys cook for another 1.5 to 2 hours until soft and done.

Quinoa (1/2-cup, cooked, 1.0 g)
Quinoa is covered in Chapter 7.

Potato (1/2-cup, cooked/mashed 0.6 to 0.8 g)
Despite the bad press, potatoes are a resistant starch, possess only 26 calories, and are packed with nutrients. Potato is rich in immune-boosting vitamin C and B, potassium, magnesium and iron. It contains a blood pressure lowering chemical called kukoamines, which the Chinese use in making teas for lowering blood pressure. And with 60 different kinds of phytochemicals and vitamins, the potato reduces the risk of cardiovascular disease and bad LDL-cholesterol and keeps arteries fat-free.

Did you know that one potato serves as 12 percent of your daily-recommended dose of fiber? They improve bowel health and support healthy digestion. Rich in vitamin B6, this tuber helps to reduce stress.

CHAPTER NINE: Read the Label

If you're recently new to the Gluten-Free diet, it can be confusing and frustrating in attempting to navigate labels. Many countries have Gluten-Free certification programs in place. If you hunt through the Gluten-Free section of your local health food store or supermarket, you'll spot the logo on products. Or ask an employee to help you identify the certification logo.

There are ingredients listed on labels that use scientific names and that mean wheat, barley, or rye and they contain gluten. So be watchful of these names.

Scientific terms for ingredients with gluten on a food label include the following:

Triticum

Triticum is a type of cultivated wheat species, generally known as the most common type of wheat called 'bread wheat.' So stay away from any labels using this word.

Triticum vulgare (wheat)

Triticale (cross between wheat and rye)

Triticum spelta (spelt, a form of wheat)

Hordeum vulgare

Hordeum vulgare is the scientific name for barley.

Secale Cereale

Secale cereale is the scientific name for rye.

Forms of Wheat, Barley, Rye

There are ingredients and processed foods that are included as a "form" of wheat, barley, and rye. They are as follows:

Bulgur (a form of wheat)
Malt (made from barley)
Couscous (made from wheat)
Farina (made from wheat)
Pasta (made from wheat unless otherwise indicated)
Seitan (made from wheat gluten and commonly used in vegetarian meals)

Wheat Starch

People with Celiac disease, wheat allergies or wheat intolerance should avoid any foods containing wheat starch. It is a powder manufactured by the removal of proteins, including gluten, from wheat flour. While most of the proteins and gluten are removed, some may still be present. People with Celiac disease have reported reactions to products containing wheat starch. This may be due to the fact that some mills may use the same machinery for processing starch and gluten. Wheat starch is used as a thickening agent and stabilizer in gravies and processed foods. Watch for the terms:

Wheat protein/hydrolyzed wheat protein
Wheat starch/hydrolyzed wheat starch

Wheat Flour

Watch out for ingredients and products containing:

Wheat flour/bread flour/bleached flour
Wheat or barley grass (will be cross contaminated)
Wheat germ oil or extract (will be cross contaminated)

Products and Ingredients that May Contain Gluten

Nowadays supermarket shelves are filled with ingredients that are produced around the world. So, it's best to check all labels to ensure your foods are free of gluten.

Some of the ingredients on this list may or may not include gluten. Be sure to check the manufacturer before consuming. Most manufacturers have websites online.

Vegetable protein/hydrolyzed protein (can come from wheat, corn or soy)
Modified starch/modified food starch (can come from wheat)
Natural flavor (can come from barley)
Modified food starch
Hydrolyzed plant protein (HPP)
Hydrolyzed vegetable protein (HVP)
Seasonings
Gravies
Vegetable starch
Dextrin and Maltodextrin (sometimes comes from wheat)

Flavorings

The terms 'natural flavor or natural flavoring' refers to the essential oil or extract of any product through roasting, heating or enzymolysis. This can be the extract from spices, fruits, vegetables, edible yeast, herbs, bark, leaves and plants. So, be careful as the 'natural flavoring' in an ingredient or product may come from a grain with gluten. Flavorings can often come from wheat and rye. Smoky flavoring comes from the burning of woods, such as mesquite or hickory. But again, be careful. Barley malt flour may be used as a carrier ingredient to help capture the aromas and flavors of the smoke.

Alcohol-Based Extracts

Alcohol based extracts like vanilla are Gluten-Free. The reason is that the alcohol in these products is distilled. Pure distilled alcohol is Gluten-Free regardless of the starting ingredient. During distillation the liquid from a fermented grain mash is boiled and the resulting byproduct is vapor. The vapor is captured and cooled and becomes liquid again. Because protein doesn't vaporize there are no proteins in the cooled liquid or extract.

Caramel

Caramel comes from cornstarch and so is Gluten-Free. Watch out for European ingredients with caramel, however. In Europe the caramel can be derived from barley or wheat.

Frozen Fruits and Vegetables

Fresh fruits and vegetables are Gluten-Free, but watch out for frozen versions. Sometimes frozen fruits and vegetables can be packaged on the same equipment or lines as wheat products. Cross contamination can be an issue. The key is to buy fresh when possible. And read labels.

Fresh meat and fish are Gluten-Free. Often in supermarkets fresh fish, poultry and meat are already seasoned. Refrain from purchasing these products. Flour is often uses as seasoning filler.

Dairy Products

Dairy products should be consumed in moderation. Not all milk and dairy-based products are Gluten-Free though. Plain milk and yogurt is Gluten-Free. But flavored versions may not be. Refrain from yogurts with granola and ice cream with cookie dough.

Cheeses are generally Gluten-Free unless they've been washed in a beer brine solution. Check with your cheese monger before purchasing.

CHAPTER TEN: Gluten-Free Tips

Shopping for Gluten-Free food can be quite difficult especially for those people who are new to this lifestyle choice. Here are some shopping tips to keep in mind while buying everyday needs that would fit into a Gluten-Free lifestyle.

Tip 1: Read the label

The most important thing a Gluten-Free dieter should do is read labels. Most food products nowadays contain an extensive list of unfamiliar looking ingredients. Make sure that when you look at the list there are no traces of wheat, barley, or rye.

Tip 2: Buy Only What You Know

Never purchase any food that you are unsure of its ingredient list. If a label isn't precise or totally clear, then contact the manufacturer and ask about their product. This way, there will be no confusion since the information will be coming from the company who actually made the product.

Tip 3: Eat Gluten-Free Processed Foods Moderately

A recent study revealed that 81% of people suffering from Celiac disease who followed a Gluten-Free diet gained weight. The reason is that there is a common misconception that "Gluten-Free" foods are healthy and low in fat. This is not necessarily the case.

Supermarkets now carry many brands of "processed" Gluten-Free foods and Gluten-Free snack foods. Some of these products can be high in fat and calories and still be Gluten-Free. Processed Gluten-Free foods are lower in fiber, so you won't stay full as long. Those who partake in a Gluten-Free diet high in processed foods miss out on all the nutrition and health benefits available from eating whole grains, fruits, vegetables and beans, which digest slowly and regulate the blood sugar.

There is a way to go Gluten-Free naturally with a diet rich in whole and unprocessed foods, fruits, vegetables, beans and lean cuts of protein.

Tip 4: Watch for hidden sources of gluten
Here are a few main culprits:

Egg Dishes, Quiche, Scrambled, and Omelets: Be careful when ordering egg-based dishes while dining out. Chefs often add flour to eggs to give quiche, scrambled eggs and omelets firmness. Be sure to ask your server about the ingredients used in the restaurant's egg-based dishes.

Sauces, Soups, Gravies and Casseroles: Be careful when dining out and indulging in classic comfort foods that incorporate 'roux.' Roux is a smooth mixture of flour and fat like bacon fat or butter. It is often used as a thickening agent in the creation of gravies, sauces and soups. Gluten can be hidden in mac and cheese, pasta with Alfredo sauce, and gravies in potpies, casseroles, gumbos, soups and stews.

Breadcrumbs in Ground Meat: When shopping, be sure to watch out for breadcrumbs used in ground meat products. Hamburger patties, meatloaf, meatballs and cabbage rolls often contain breadcrumbs. (You can make your own Gluten-Free Panko breadcrumbs by placing about 3 cups of Rice Chex Cereal in a plastic bag and rolling a pin over them to make coarse or fine crumbs.)

Vitamins, dietary supplements and pharmaceutical drugs: Gluten can be hidden and used as filler in vitamins, supplements and drugs.

Chinese Food: Unfortunately, some of the tastiest sauces used in Chinese cuisine have gluten, such as soy, fish, oyster and bean sauces. They contain wheat. If craving Chinese food, you may have to make it yourself.

For the estimated three million Americans suffering from Celiac disease, wheat allergies, and severe gluten sensitivities, Asian food is usually off-limits because its signature ingredients— noodles, soy sauce, and oyster sauce—typically contain wheat. In the *Gluten-Free Asian Kitchen*, food writer Laura B. Russell shows home cooks how to convert the vibrant cuisines of China, Japan, Korea, Thailand, and Vietnam into Gluten-Free favorites. Authentically flavored dishes such as Crispy Spring Rolls, Gingery Pork Pot Stickers, Korean Green Onion Pancakes, Soba Noodles with Stir-Fried Shiitake Mushrooms, Salt and Pepper Squid, and Pork Tonkatsu will be delicious additions to any Gluten-Free repertoire. Along with sharing approachable and delicious recipes, Russell demystifies Asian ingredients and helps readers navigate the grocery store. Beautifully photographed and designed for easy weeknight eating, this unique cookbook's wide range of dishes from a variety of Asian cuisines will appeal to the discriminating tastes of today's Gluten-Free cooks.

Tip 5: French fries.

While classic fries use only potatoes, seasoned versions incorporate flour. So watch out when dining out. Also be aware that even when the fries have not been coated, the deep frying oils can be still be contaminated with breading from other foods.

Tip 6: Kitchen appliances.

Your toaster and baking-oven maybe a hotbed of gluten residue. While this does not affect me in being gluten-sensitive, it is vital for those with gluten intolerance or Celiac disease.

Tip 7: Diet soda, artificially sweetened foods.

Aspartame is recognized as a serious offender for those with a gluten intolerance or Celiac disease. It can trigger similar allergic symptoms, such as stomach pain and bloating.

CHAPTER ELEVEN: Speeding Up Your Metabolism

We know that weight loss is closely associated with our metabolism. What exactly is metabolism?

Metabolism is the amount of energy or calories our bodies need to maintain throughout the day. Everyone's metabolism is different and is affected by their body composition. People with greater muscle mass will have a higher metabolism. Those with less muscle have a slower one.

Those with greater muscle mass can consume more calories without gaining weight. Probably one of the most effective ways to speed up the metabolism is to exercise regularly incorporating both aerobic and anaerobic exercise, such as weight lifting.

The good news is that there are a few tips and ingredients and foods that you can incorporate into your Gluten-Free diet to speed up your metabolism.

Tip 1: Exercise moderately and regularly:
Throughout my teens, 20's and 30's I was obsessed with staying thin, depriving myself of food, binge eating and working out like a maniac. When I hit my 40's and remarried and found happiness, I went in the opposite direction. I gave up exercise, ate and drank whatever I enjoyed and gained an enormous amount of weight. Now in my 50's I've finally found moderation. I have found a few girlfriends who also enjoy walking. This is so I am not tied to the schedule of just one person. I walk but 3 miles on each outing, and do this consistently. It is the consistency of my moderate walking that has contributed toward the shedding of my extra weight. On good days my girlfriend and I will walk faster, not longer.

Tip 2: Drink Less Alcohol:

As a food and wine writer, it's important that I recipe test and assess wines for my column. I enjoy a glass of wine with my meals -- sometimes 2 glasses. But I no longer drink wine every day. I assess wines, that is smell and taste them and then spittoon – spit them out. I now "drink" wine on occasion. Regular alcohol consumption is detrimental to weight loss. Alcohol stimulates the appetite causing us to eat more food during the meal. It also adds calories and slows the metabolism.

Tip 3: Sleep at least 7 to 8 hours per night:
The timing, duration, and quality of our sleep directly affect endocrine, metabolic, and neurohormonal functions related to our health. Proper sleep is vital in the control and management of our weight. Getting proper sleep decreases the risk of metabolic disorders such as insulin resistance and diabetes, to name but two.

Research also now reveals a link between our metabolism and sleep. Not getting enough sleep can slow one's metabolism. The quality of your sleep also orchestrates a symphony of hormonal activity tied to your appetite. Research on the hormones called leptin and ghrelin show that both can influence our appetite. And studies show that production of both may be influenced by how much or how little we sleep. Have you ever experienced a sleepless night and the next day your hunger never seems to be satisfied? This is a result of leptin and ghrelin at work.

Tip 4: Adding BCAA Powder to your shake.
BCAA stands for branched-chain amino acids. They can help repair and build muscle even when you can't make it to the gym! Muscle burns at least three times the number of calories as fat. This makes building muscle a priority for boosting the metabolism. BCAA supports your body repair and rebuilds muscle. Add 1000 mg of BCAA powder to your morning shake. Always consult your doctor before starting a new supplement to your diet.

Tip 5: Add cayenne pepper to your Gluten-Free dishes.

Cayenne contains capsaicin, a compound that stimulates the body's pain receptors, temporarily increasing blood circulation and metabolic rate. Studies have shown that eating hot peppers or cayenne can actually boost the metabolism for up to 3 hours and by up to 25%. Adding capsaicin to your diet is also healthy. Capsaicin acts as a blood thinner, helping to prevent blood clots, which reduces the incidence of blood clotting related diseases. It is also an anti-inflammatory.

Tip 6: Eat Broccoli:

Broccoli is extraordinarily high in vitamins C, K and A. One serving of this green super food also provides the body with lots of folate and dietary fiber and antioxidants. Broccoli detoxifies the body, thus helping it function more efficiently and ultimately supporting weight loss.

Tip 7: Eat Apples and Pears:

State University of Rio de Janeiro research showed that women who ate three small apples or pears daily lost more weight than those who did not.

Tip 8: Eat calcium-rich foods:

Studies show that people who consume 1200 to 130 milligrams of calcium per day lost almost double the amount of weight than those who did not. Calcium-rich foods speed the metabolism. Calcium is also necessary for the grown and maintenance of our teeth and bones, nerve signaling, muscle contraction and the secretion of certain hormones and enzymes. Foods high in calcium include:

Calcium-rich foods to incorporate into your Gluten-Free diet include:

Dark leafy greens (kale, spinach, watercress, arugula, mustard greens)
Low fat cheeses – partly skimmed mozzarella

Low to no fat yogurt
Chinese cabbage (bok choy)
Okra
Broccoli
Green snap beans
Almonds
Canned sardines
Flaxseeds
Sesame seeds
Rhubarb
Fresh parsley, thyme, basil
Garlic
Note: Be careful about taking calcium supplements. Too much calcium can lead to kidney stones, strokes and heart attacks. It's always best to attain vitamins and minerals through the foods we eat.

Tip 9: Eat foods high in Omega-3's:
Munching on foods high in omega-3 acids is the greatest way to speed up the metabolism. These acids reduce the production of a hormone called leptin, a chemical that slows the metabolism. Consume foods high in Omega-3 acids, such as nuts and seeds, hemp oil, flax seed oil, etc.

Tip 10: Consume Coconut oil:
From a medicinal standpoint, coconut oil is a super food. It is a rich source of good saturated fat with almost 90% of the fatty acids in it being saturated. The saturated fat contains Medium Chain Triglycerides (MCTs).

Every time you eat, the process of digesting food burns off at least 10 percent of the calories you consume. Try replacing fats with coconut oil and you will speed up your metabolism by 15%. That may not seem like much, but will make a difference over time. It has to do with coconut oil's molecular structure and how the body digests it. The medium chain triglycerides (MCTs) in coconut oil are shorter and more water soluble than in other oils like canola or olive oil.

The body processes coconut oil immediately and therefore there is less opportunity for the body to store it as fat. For this reason it boosts the metabolic rate.

Coconut oil can be used in shakes, salad dressings, as a butter substitute and in cooking and baking. Be sure to invest in organic cold pressed coconut oil.

I try to use this oil as a substitute for other oils in as many ways as I can. I add it to Indian and Thai-based curry, in homemade Gluten-Free banana bread, and vinaigrettes.

As an aside, I mix coconut oil with vitamin E and use it as a face and body moisturizer.

Tip 11: Eat avocados:
This creamy green fruit is high in the right fats, the monounsaturated ones, which help control the metabolic rate. It is also high in fiber, vitamins and minerals. On a daily basis and ask a snack I enjoy a dip combining avocado with fat free yogurt and eat it with raw vegetables.

Tip 12: Eat more soup:
Research shows that flavorful soup satisfies both our palate and stomach, providing a combination of liquid and solid foods. Soup (those without saturated fats) can speed up the metabolism and help the body burn fat.

Tip 13: Drink purified water:
A Germany study showed that drinking water speeds up the fat burning process. It also detoxifies the body, making it more efficient to burn fat and suppresses the appetite.

Tip 14: Have a cup of caffeinated coffee:
The caffeine in coffee speeds up the heart rate, which in turn boosts the metabolism for about 3 hours. An 8-ounce cup of coffee has about 100 milligrams of caffeine. You should not consume more than 300 milligrams of caffeine per day. And you

should consult your doctor if you have any health or heart issues that could be affected by caffeine.

Keep in mind that dark coffees are not necessarily stronger in caffeine. The caffeine level is determined by the bean variety, bean roasting level and coffee making process.

Robusto coffee beans have double the amount of caffeine than Arabica.

Lighter roasted coffees have more caffeine than darker roasts. This is because the prolonged toasting or heating of the beans breaks down the caffeine molecules.

The grind and the brewing process also affect the level of caffeine in the coffee.

The longer the coffee is brewed, the higher the level of its caffeine. French pressed coffee has a higher caffeine level because it is left to sit for a longer period of time.

So espresso, while stronger tasting, has less caffeine than brewed coffee.

Tip 15: Drink tea:
I am addicted to tea, almost as much as to wine. In fact, in an effort to lose weight, I cut back tremendously on wine sipping and replaced the habit with sipping tea – all kinds of tea. I crave the tannin in black tea as it has helped to subside my craving for the tannin in red wine. It has helped tremendously.

True tea is made from the leaves of an Asian evergreen known as Camellia sinensis. White tea, green tea, oolong tea, and black tea all derive from this plant. They also contain caffeine and so speed up the metabolism. Many factors influence how much caffeine is present in plucked tea leaves, such as the growing region, plant variety, age, leaf-age, nutrients, rainfall and stress by pests. The final production of the leaves from plant to tea also affects the level of caffeine.

The entire tea preparing process also affects its caffeine level. The temperature of the water used, brewing time and whether the leaves are loose, bagged or strained, also play an important role in the tea's caffeine level.

Tea Variety and Caffeine Level per 8 Ounce Cup
- White tea; 30 to 55 mg
- Green tea; 35 to 70 mg
- Oolong tea; 50 to 75 mg
- Black tea; 60 to 90 mg

Tip 16: Drink Green Tea:
Green tea is often an ingredient in weight loss products because it has been proven to burn fat and calories and speed up the metabolism. It also proves endurance during exercise. Green tea contains epiogallocatechin 3-gallate, a powerful antioxidant that stimulates the metabolism and enhances fat burning.

In the human body high levels of triglycerides in the bloodstream have been linked to heart disease and strokes. Triglyceride is a very important substance, because it provides energy to support various functions of the body. Diets high in refined carbohydrates can increase triglyceride levels. Excess triglyceride can be transformed into fat, which can result in obesity. Drinking great tea on a regular basis will help to reduce the fat in your body.

Tip 17: Eat papaya
Papaya contains papain, an enzyme that improves protein digestion and absorption. This is key to boosting metabolism and burning fat. Try incorporating this exotic super food into your diet. It can be added to salads, baked goods, desserts, dressings, salsa and sauces.

Conclusion

I really want to thank you for reading this book. I sincerely hope my words have provided value for you and make a difference for you in your life. If you did receive value from this book, I would like to ask a favor of you. (Know that you also have the right to decline this request.)

Would you be kind enough to leave a review for my book on Amazon.com?

If so please click the link below to leave a review.

http://understandpublishing.com/visit/love-your-review/

The End